A Practical Guide to Treating Eczema in Children

Dr James Halpern

Consultant Dermatologist

Introduction

Eczema can be a devastating condition, yet friends, family and even healthcare professionals dismiss it. How many times do you hear others say *it is only eczema.* Yet they are wrong, eczema ruins lives. Your child is suffering, they are not sleeping, you are not sleeping. Everywhere you turn there is different advice – it is food allergy, it is a clothes allergy, use steroids, don't use steroids. The internet, health professionals and book shops are full of often contradictory advice of what to do. Why is this book any different?

I am a doctor who has spent my career specialising in and treating children with eczema. I am also a father of two children with eczema. As much as I have learned from my professional career it is only since having my own children that I have truly understood how overwhelming eczema can be. This book balances the professional 'ideal' ways of treating eczema against the practicalities of doing this in real life. There are hints, tips and practical solutions to everyday situations and answers to all the commonest questions parents ask me.

This book is purposefully short and pragmatic, so it can be read quickly and the eczema can be treated properly as soon as possible. If you follow the advice in this book your child will get better and they will stay better. It may not be easy but you will be amazed how much better your child can be and how much this will improve your life.

Dr James Halpern MBChB, BMedSci, MRCP(UK)(Dermatology), FRCP Ed
Consultant Dermatologist

Index

What is Eczema?

Key points

- In eczema the skin becomes red, dry, itchy, sore and sensitive
- Eczema is a chronic condition and it cannot be cured
- By using the right treatments eczema can be treated, but if treatment is stopped eczema will come back
- Eczema is very common
- Most grow out of eczema
- No one really knows what causes eczema and it is likely to be a mixture of many different factors
- Eczema has a massive effect on the whole family having a similar impact as conditions such as epilepsy or diabetes

Basic facts about eczema

Eczema is a condition of which affects the skin. What starts as 'sensitive skin' and dryness develops into a cycle of progressive inflammation. This inflamed skin is red, sore, dry and itchy. Unfortunately there is no cure for eczema, it is chronic condition that lasts for many years and in a small number of cases it lasts for life. There are effective treatments for eczema and when these are used properly the inflammation is suppressed and skin returns to normal. It is though vital that treatment is maintained as if it is stopped the eczema will return. As part of the normal eczema condition it will go through cycles of flaring and settling. I have seen parents driving themselves mad trying to find out what is triggering the flares, when in the majority of cases there simply is no trigger.

It is an extremely common condition with one in five of all children suffering from it. The majority of children only have it mildly whilst others suffer from extremely severe disease. Although it is confusing dermatitis means the same as eczema, it is two names for the same condition and the terms are used interchangeably. Eczema is not an infectious condition, your child has not caught it and they cannot give it to anyone else. When someone in the household has an itchy skin condition it is normal for other member of the family to feel itchy, this is a psychological response, no one has caught eczema. Eczema does not scar, this is understandably of great concern to parents and relatives especially when the eczema is severe. It does not though ever cause scarring and when children with even severe eczema grow out of their condition they have normal, unblemished skin. The only exception to this is deep scratches of the skin which may scar and this is one of the reasons why it is so important to treat the eczema and prevent this. Perhaps most importantly there is light at the end of the tunnel, if used properly treated is effective in nearly all cases of eczema and the vast majority of children grow out of eczema as they get older.

At what age does eczema occur?

Eczema can occur at any age and I see it in babies appearing at or soon after birth right up to people in their mid-nineties presenting with eczema for the first time. Most commonly though, eczema occurs in children with over ninety percent of eczema appearing before the age of five years. In most cases children do eventually grow out of their eczema, about half of all children with eczema grow out of it by six years of age. Most of the rest will grow out of their eczema in their early teenage years. There are only a few children in which the eczema continues on into adulthood. In my experience children who develop eczema as a young baby tend to grow out of it earlier than those who develop it as a toddler. If a child still has eczema as they are coming to the end of school it becomes less likely that they will grow out of it.

What causes eczema

There are different types of eczema and the cause of the eczema depends on the type. For example a machine worker who is constantly exposing his hands to oils may get an eczema on their hands due to the direct irritation of the skin by the oil. This is called an irritant eczema. Another example would be someone with a hair dye allergy developing an eczema of their scalp after having their hair treated. This is an allergic type of eczema called allergic contact dermatitis.

In children the vast majority of eczema is atopic eczema and this is due to atopy. Atopy is a genetically inherited condition which means it tends to run in families and other close relatives are also likely to have it. Having atopy means children are more likely to develop a number of conditions such as eczema, asthma, hayfever, hives and allergies. It is not though always the case that relatives have atopy and a child may be the first in the family to develop eczema, this is particularly common in second generation immigrants.

When children have atopy a number of different things are happening which leads them to develop atopic eczema. Primarily there is damage to the natural layer of oil that protects the skin. All people produce natural oils that moisturise the skin and protect it. In eczema this protective layer is damaged, moisture leaks out, irritant chemicals are let in and the skin becomes dry and inflamed. One of the reasons we use moisturisers to treat eczema is to replace and repair the skins own natural oily protective barrier. In addition to this there are very complicated changes to the body's immune system that we do not fully understand. These changes cause to skin to overreact when exposed to infections, allergens, heat and irritation. This causes redness, inflammation and soreness. Steroid ointments work by dampening down this overreaction of the immune system.

Once children have eczema there are a number of things that can make it worse and cause flares. Most commonly though it is just part of the eczema. Eczema naturally goes through phases of being settled and flaring, similar to how a child with asthma will have 'good weeks' and 'bad weeks' for no obvious reason.

The impact of eczema on the whole family

Eczema is an incredibly frustrating condition; it has a massive impact on the child and the family but is often dismissed by family, friends and even healthcare professionals. How many times do parents hear the phrase 'it is only eczema', this is not only upsetting but it compounds the problem by making you feel that you are a failure for not coping with it. You need to tell yourself that people aren't being dismissive; they simply fail to understand how much of an impact the eczema is having on your life. As eczema is so common, the majority of cases are mild and easily treated, giving an impression to some people that all cases are like this. The fact that you are reading this book is a testament to show that your child does not have simple, easy to treat eczema and you are trying your hardest to help them.

I often see a cycle of despair developing in families of children with uncontrolled eczema. The child with eczema is uncomfortable and sleeping poorly, because of this the child is on-edge, emotionally fragile and quick to cry. The parents, who themselves are sleep deprived and emotionally strained are then trying their best to look after often a very difficult and unhappy child. This leads to a devastating effect on the whole family with everyone being stressed, unhappy and sleep deprived.

Research has been done looking at children with severe eczema and how their illness affects the life of the child and their family. It was shown that their quality of life is impaired as much as children with other serious chronic medical problems such as epilepsy, kidney disease and diabetes.

There is though hope, with the right treatment a child's eczema can be controlled and as the child feels better they sleep better, they are happier and life becomes better for the whole family. The cycle of eczema and its impact on the family can be broken and key to this having the right treatment, doing the treatment correctly and continuing on with treatment.

Types of eczema

Key points

- There are lots of types of eczema
- Different types of eczema present in different ways and look different
- Treatment may also be different depending on the type of eczema
- Some types of eczema are hard to diagnose and may mimic other skin conditions such as psoriasis and fungal infections
- As children get older the type of eczema they have may change
- It is important to know what type of eczema your child has so they can get the best treatment

Atopic eczema

Nearly all children with eczema have atopic eczema which is also known as atopic dermatitis; this is sometimes referred to as normal, typical or common eczema. The different types of eczema described below are all forms of atopic eczema. Atopy and how it causes eczema is discussed in the previous chapter. Eczema not due to atopy is very rare in children and is discussed later.

Infantile eczema

Babies may develop eczema at or soon after birth. When children develop eczema under one year of age they often present with infantile eczema. This type of eczema is red and dry, there are often small scratch marks the baby's nails. It is most commonly seen on the face, especially the cheeks and can become widespread covering much of the body. This type of eczema is rarely present on the bottom and if it is present it is often mild in this area. Saying this, like all children they can develop nappy rash. As these children become toddlers the eczema changes and turns into extensor eczema and then flexural eczema.

Extensor eczema

Toddlers often present with extensor eczema, this type of eczema tends to affect children aged between two and four years of age. Infantile eczema which is thin and widespread becomes localised to areas on the skin and starts to thicken. It tends to affect the front of the knees and shin, around the wrists, the ankles and the outside of the elbows. At this age toddlers tend to scratch the eczema a lot leaving lots of marks. The thick, scratched, often dark patches of eczema are referred to by the medical name lichenified. The thicker patches often require a step up the strength of steroid ointments to treat them.

Flexural eczema

As children get older extensor eczema develops into flexural eczema, which is the most common type of eczema seen. This change tends to occur around four years of age. Children who develop eczema for the first time at this age also tend to present with flexural eczema. Like in extensor eczema the rash is localised and can become thickened. It moves to the body creases such as the back of the knee, the inside of the elbows and around the neck. When it occurs around the neck the skin can darken and give a permanently dirty look, this is called an atopic dirty neck and is a sign of eczema. Once this pattern of eczema has established it tends to stay in this distribution until the child grows out of it, or continue with this pattern into adulthood.

Discoid eczema

Discoid eczema is also known by the names nummular dermatitis and microbial eczema, these are all different names for the same condition. This type of eczema is more common in adults but it is also seen in some children. The eczema occurs as round or oval patches from one to ten centimeters in diameter. The patches are often thickened and may be weepy, they are most common on the arms and legs but may appear anywhere on the body. This type of eczema is often misdiagnosed as a fungal infection of the skin. The conditions can be distinguished as fungal infections are not itchy and they tend to have a clear area of normal skin in the middle of the patch, unlike discoid eczema which is very itchy and the whole patch is filled in with eczema. This type of eczema often requires stronger treatments than other types of eczema. There is also an infective component to this type of eczema and creams mixed with antiseptics or antibiotics can be helpful.

Seborrhoeic dermatitis

Seborrhoeic dermatitis is a type of eczema that can affect children and adults of any age. It most commonly presents as a scaly scalp. In children the scaly scalp is called cradle cap and the scale is often thickened and greasy. In adults the scaly scalp is called dandruff and the scale is light and dry. In more severe cases babies, often under six months of age, have a widespread greasy looking eczema alongside cradle cap. As children get older the eczema localises to the central chest, ears and the sides of the nose. This type of eczema is partly due to the overgrowth of a harmless yeast that lives on all of our skins. Antifungal and coal tar preparations are used to treat seborrhoeic dermatitis as they are effective at killing off the yeast.

Pompholyx eczema

Pompholyx eczema is also known by the name dishydrotic eczema, these are two names for the same condition. Although this is more common in adults it is seen people of all ages including children. This type of eczema affects the hands and feet, particularly the palms, soles, fingers and toes. Initially patients develop hundreds of tiny, clear, fluid filled blisters just under the skin. These may vary between being intensely itchy and not itchy at all. In time the skin on the hands and feet in more severe cases becomes dry, cracked and fissured. Often this type of eczema comes and goes and tends to appear at the change of seasons in the spring and autumn. Pompholyx eczema may occur in isolation or be associated with other types of eczema. Often quite strong steroid creams are required to treat this type of eczema.

Juvenile plantar dermatosis

Juvenile plantar dermatosis is a special type of eczema that most commonly affects young boys. It is more common in children who have atopy and atopic eczema. It affects the sole of the foot over the balls of the feet and the toes. The skin becomes shiny, glazed and can crack. It is often worse in the summer and when it is hot. It is thought that the condition is caused by the feet becoming sweaty and rubbing against the bottom of the shoe. Trainers and plastic shoes that do not let the feet 'breathe' are largely responsible and changing to leather shoes helps the problem.

Non-atopic eczema

Eczema not due to atopy is rare in children although two types are seen, allergic contact dermatitis and irritant contact dermatitis.

Allergic contact dermatitis is a form of allergy where a compound placed on the skin induces a patch of eczema. The commonest example of this is people who cannot tolerate costume jewelry and must wear gold or silver. This is due to allergy to nickel, a silver coloured metal that is present in cheap jewelry, jean buttons and belts. In this case unusual patches of eczema appear in places such as the earlobes where earrings are worn, under watch straps and on the lower abdomen next to buttons. Another example often seen in adults is allergy to a chemical that is often present in hair dyes. It is rare for eczema in children to caused by allergic contact dermatitis but when this is suspected they can be tested with a type of allergy testing known as patch testing. Blood tests are not helpful in this type of allergy.

Irritant contact dermatitis is a type of eczema caused by chronic irritation of the skin by an irritant compound which breaks the skin down into eczema. A common example of this is children who suck their thumbs, where the combination of mechanical irritation of the skin and saliva break down the surface of the skin into eczema. Another example of this is Lip Licking Dermatitis where children constantly lick the skin surrounding the lips causing eczema to appear in an unusual ring around the mouth. Nappy rash is also a type of irritant eczema. It is also known by the medical name napkin dermatitis. It is more common in children with sensitive skin and eczema. It is due to the nappy contents which sit against the skin causing irritation. Eventually the skin becomes so irritated that it develops into an eczema. In severe cases the skin can break down causing open sores and small ulcers.

Hand dermatitis

Hand dermatitis is a type of eczema that affects the hands; it may also affect the feet when it is known as hand and foot dermatitis. It most commonly affects the palms of the hand the sides of the fingers with a dry, red, inflamed eczema that can crack leaving deep fissures. This is a particularly chronic form of eczema that is difficult to treat. It is also unusual as it may be caused by atopy, irritant contact dermatitis or allergic contact dermatitis. Often it is due to a combination of all three of these causes of eczema. Treatment involves using frequent moisturisers, strong steroid ointments and avoiding irritants such as soap and cleaning products.

Eczema in Pigmented Skin

Key points

- In different ethnic groups eczema acts differently
- When eczema occurs in darker skin types it often leaves patches of colour change on the skin
- Most commonly light patches of skin are seen on the face known as Pityriasis Alba
- Some types of eczema are more common in darker skin and different treatments may be needed
- Eczema often improves when travelling to hot countries
- Healthcare professionals in predominantly white areas are sometimes caught out by eczema in pigmented skin

Colour change

When seeing children with eczema and pigmented (dark) skin the question I am asked most often asked about is colour change. In white skin when a patch of eczema is treated and goes the skin left behind looks normal. In children with brown or black coloured skin when a patch of eczema goes it often leaves an area of skin with changed colour. This is very common and I see it in nearly all children I look after of South Asian or Afro-Caribbean descent.

The colour change is due to inflammation in the skin, in this case the inflammation is due to eczema. Similar colour changes also occur in other skin conditions that inflame the skin such as psoriasis. The colour change may present as lightening of the skin colour, medically this is called Post-inflammatory hypopigmentation. It may also present as darkening of the skin colour, this is called Post-inflammatory hyperpigmentation. In some children they have a mixture with both dark and light patches of skin.

Sometimes parents worry that the colour change is due to the steroid creams given to treat the eczema. This is almost never the case, the steroids given as creams are simply not strong enough to cause bleaching of the skin. The colour change is due to the inflammation caused by active eczema. In fact using steroid creams will dampen down the inflammation and stop the colour change getting any worse. There are no effective treatments for the colour change other than treating the eczema well and waiting. Occasionally parents try to use bleaching creams to lighten the darker patches; this flares the eczema making the patch even darker and must be avoided.

Skin colour change with eczema is not a form of scarring and is not permanent. As children grow up and the eczema settles the colour change will also go. It is often a slow process and it may take a number of years for the skin to return to its normal colour. It does though always return to normal and your child will have a normal colour to their skin when they grow up.

Pityriasis alba

A related condition to eczema which I am often asked to see in children with pigmented skin is Pityriasis alba. It occurs in children with eczema and also in children who have sensitive skin that has not yet broken out into eczema. It presents as light patches of skin on the face, most commonly on the cheeks. It may be symmetrical and the edges of the colour change are not crisp or well defined. Pityriasis alba is caused by the same process as eczema related colour change and is a type of post-inflammatory hypopigmentation. Unlike in eczema it can occur spontaneously and often there is no visible eczema prior to the colour changing.

Understandably parents get very worried about Pityriasis alba, particularly as it is on the face and is obvious. Their main worries are that it will get worse, spread and be permanent. Like with eczema related colour change it is only temporary and as children grow up it completely resolves leaving no marks behind. It also tends to remain a mild colour change and never goes completely white.

Sometimes health professionals don't know about Pityriasis alba and misdiagnose it as a fungal infection or a separate skin condition called Vitiligo. Fortunately fungal infections of the face are rare and are normally given away by the edge of the patch of colour change being scaly, the centre of a fungal infection is also normally spared giving a ring appearance which is not present in Pityriasis alba. In Vitiligo the area of colour change is completely white rather than being a lighter shade of the normal skin colour. A simple test to distinguish Vitiligo from Pityriasis alba is to hold a piece of white writing paper next to the skin. If the skin is as white as the paper then it is more likely to be vitiligo, if the skin is a light brown then it is more likely to be Pityriasis alba.

Treatment of Pityriasis alba is with moisturisers. If there is no active eczema visible then steroid creams are not needed. Children with Pityriasis alba are at risk of developing eczema and their skin should be treated with care. They should be moisturised twice daily and avoid putting soaps, shampoos and bubble baths on the skin.

First children in the family with eczema

Often the first generations of children born to families who have emigrated are the first in the family to develop eczema. This makes it particularly hard as no one else in the family has experience of eczema and can give advice and support. No one really knows why this happens although there are a number of theories and it is something I see a lot.

The most likely reason is differences in climate, particularly sunshine and altitude. We know that sunshine is an effective treatment for eczema, often children with eczema find that if they go on a sunny holiday the eczema improves. Dermatologists even use sunlight as a treatment for people with severe eczema, this is called phototherapy. It is likely that lots of children in hot countries have eczema, but as it is always treated by the sunshine and it never appears on the skin. In a similar manner when children with eczema go on holiday to their family countries of origin the eczema is treated by the sun and improves.

Another theory is that the difference is due to house dust mite. House dust mite is a tiny insect that lives in soft furnishings such as carpets and beds. In hot countries house dust mite is much less common as they do not like the heat and there tends to be less soft furnishings for the insect to live in. Nearly all children with eczema are allergic to house dust mite and it is theorised that this may be one reason why children in northern developed countries are more likely to develop eczema. Interestingly though there is little evidence that reducing house dust mite levels in western countries improves eczema.

Eczema differences in pigmented skin

Eczema is different in children with darker skin colour, it looks different, behaves differently and may need different treatment. This is often a challenge for health professionals who work in predominantly Caucasian areas and have little experience in treating eczema in pigmented skin.

As well as the obvious difference in colour in pigmented skin there are also differences in skin structure, structural proteins which make up the skin and the immune system. The most commonly seen difference in pigmented skin is the colour changes that eczema causes as discussed above. Dark thick patches of eczema are seen that may mimic other skin disorders and be hard to diagnose. This type of eczema often needs stronger steroid ointments to treat it than would normally be used. Some of the less common types of eczema such as discoid eczema are also more common in pigmented skin and in black skin eczema can be very dry. Normal cream based moisturisers are often ineffective and greasy, ointment based preparations are required.

Moisturisers

Key points

- Moisturisers are oil based products that are applied to skin to treat dry skin and eczema

- Moisturisers are also known as emollients

- They are the corner stone of treating all forms and severities of eczema

- There are different types of moisturiser and it is important to know which moisturisers to use for which forms of eczema

- Certain moisturisers seem to suit particular children and parents may need to try a few different products before finding one which suits their child's skin

- Parents and health professionals often underestimate the amount of moisturisers needed

- It is safe to apply as much moisturiser as you want, as frequently as you want to

- Some parents find it helpful to use two or more different moisturisers

- True allergy to moisturisers is very rare

How moisturisers work

Eczema is a condition where the bodies own natural protective oily skin layer has broken down, this makes the skin dry and inflamed as it loses moisture. By applying moisturisers you are both giving a temporarily replacement for this and helping to repair the body's own natural oily layer. Additionally moisturisers act as a protective layer blocking irritant compounds and allergens from reaching the skin itself. They also directly hydrate and treat dry areas of skin by attracting moisture from the air.

The majority of moisturisers are an emulsion which is a mixture of oil and water. The proportion of oil to water and which type of oil is used will determine the texture of the moisturiser, how thick it is and how easy it is to rub in. Some moisturisers use thin oils similar to petrol which have a similar consistency to water, others use thick oils which have solidified such as paraffin. Some of the very thick moisturisers are composed entirely of oils with no water. Other chemicals are often added to enhance the moisturising ability or directly replace lipids that have been lost from the skin.

As well as treating eczema moisturisers are widely marketed in the cosmetic industry to treat wrinkles and age related skin problems. This type of moisturiser should be avoided in eczema as they often contain additional chemicals and fragrances that children with eczema may be allergic to.

How to moisturise the skin

It is important that moisturisers are applied to all of the skin on the body, not just to the areas affected by eczema. This will prevent new areas of eczema occurring by keeping the unaffected skin well hydrated and suppressing any inflammation. Even if a child's eczema has completely disappeared moisturisers should be applied regularly to all of the skin to prevent the eczema coming back.

Moisturisers are completely safe and there is no such thing as moisturising too much. In fact the more you moisturise the better, the commonest cause of eczema flaring is not moisturising enough. The moisturiser should be applied at least twice a day although ideally more frequently than this. Unfortunately there is a tendency for health professionals to underestimate how much moisturiser children with eczema require and to not prescribe enough of it. Most moisturisers can and should be prescribed in large 500g or 1kg containers, the smaller 100g tubes should only be prescribed for portability and used when out and about. There is no place for using tubes of cream smaller than 100g as they will be used up too quickly. If you are covering your child in moisturiser properly twice a day you should be using between 250g and 500g of moisturiser a week. This amount is often a shock to parents who often use much smaller amounts than this.

Applying moisturisers and steroid creams is very time consuming and you should set aside at least half an hour each morning and each evening for applying the creams. As a parent you should be applying the creams to your child personally and not leaving it to others. However mature your child they are very unlikely to apply enough of the creams and apply them properly. Teachers also do not have the time or training to apply the creams. When applying moisturisers they should be spread in the direction of hair growth on the skin, this is to reduce the chance of blocking hair follicles and it is particularly important when using thicker, greasy moisturisers. Nearly all moisturisers can also be used as soap substitutes and this is discussed further in the chapter on bathing.

It is important to know that thick ointment based moisturisers have high concentrations of paraffin which is flammable. It is important to avoid naked flames, electric heaters and cigarettes around children using these products.

A note on aqueous cream

The use of aqueous cream as a leave on moisturiser is controversial. I would not personally recommend the usage of this product although I am aware of a small number of children who do use it and find it helpful.

Aqueous cream was originally designed as a soap substitute and meant to be washed off the skin after use. It was never intended to be rubbed into the skin and used as a leave on moisturiser. The product is manufactured by a number of different companies each with slightly different recipes. This means that one tub of aqueous cream may be substantially different from another tub and you don't really know what you are putting on your child's skin.

Many preparations of aqueous cream contain a chemical called sodium lauryl sulphate. This is damaging to the skin in a number of ways including raising the pH and making it alkaline. There are now some preparations of aqueous cream available without sodium lauryl sulphate. In the past few years there has been good published research showing that aqueous cream damages the skin in people predisposed to eczema rather than helping it. In my practice I have found that switching from aqueous cream to other products can make a substantial improvement to a child's eczema.

Which moisturiser should I use?

The simple answer to this question, is the moisturiser that most suits your child's skin. Through experience I have noticed that certain children seem to respond to particular moisturisers. Often there is nothing which can predict which moisturiser will suit your child best and it is a case of trying different products until you find the best one. Your healthcare professional should be able to advise on which moisturisers are likely to suit your child's skin and they may be able to supply you with sample pots for you to try.

Sometimes I see parents who have been through tens of moisturisers and tell me that none of them suit their child. In general all moisturisers will benefit children with eczema and if none are working you have to question if you are applying the creams correctly and giving them a chance to work. It is important to try each moisturiser for at least two weeks and use it properly to determine how effective it is. Additionally when contemplating a switch try and identify what it is about the current product that is not working for your child. Is it too greasy? Not greasy enough? Does it sting when it goes on? Does it leave the skin looking too shiny? Knowing this information will guide you and your health professional over which product to try next.

Another issue I am asked about are children who simply refuse to use certain moisturisers. Often this is because the child is given a thick ointment moisturiser which is good for their eczema, but they refuse to use it because it leaves the skin looking shiny and they find it hard to rub in. In these situations it is better to give a less effective thinner moisturiser which the child can use during the day and they can apply a thick moisturiser before bed to soak in overnight. Compliance with moisturising treatment is very important and it is better for a child to use a thinner moisturiser frequently and properly rather than trying a thick moisturiser which they simply won't use.

Types of moisturiser

There are a huge range of moisturisers and they vary from being very thin like a liquid through to very thick near solid preparations. There are advantages and disadvantages to the different preparations which I will discuss below. When using moisturisers it is often a balancing act between effectiveness and cosmetic acceptability and it can be helpful for a child to have multiple different moisturisers to use in different situations. A good example of this would be a teenager who uses a gel based moisturiser during the day when they do not want their skin to look shiny and an ointment based moisturiser at night when sleeping. Thicker ointment based moisturisers are the most effective but also the least cosmetically acceptable.

An added challenge is that certain brands of moisturiser can come in different preparations making it hard for parents to know what they are using. An example is a well known brand of moisturiser called Aveeno®; Aveeno® itself is not a single moisturiser but a range of products including a cream, lotion and a bath oil. Often when I see patients they tell me that they are using Aveeno® as a moisturiser but they don't know if it is the cream or the lotion. It is therefore important for parents to know not only the name of the moisturiser but also which formulation they are using. If in doubt always bring the moisturisers with you to any consultations with a health professional.

Lotions

Lotions are very thin moisturisers with a high water content that are very easy to rub in and don't leave any shine on the skin. In general they are poor at hydrating the skin and are not very effective moisturisers. In children with established, dry eczema they should be avoided except in certain situations. Lotions are useful in hairy areas as they do not block hair follicles or stick the hair together. They can also be useful in weepy forms of eczema such as pompholyx as they dry up the skin. They also have a cooling effect and can be used for symptomatic relief of particularly inflamed eczema alongside a thicker moisturiser. Lotions do tend to make good soap substitutes and are good to wash with in the bath or shower. Examples of available lotions include Aveeno® lotion, E45® lotion and QV® lotion.

Gels

Gels are similar to lotions, they have a high water content, are easy to rub in and don't leave any shine on the skin. Like lotions they are not as effective at moisturising the skin as the thicker preparations and should be avoided in very dry eczema. They are though useful in children who refuse to use the thicker products, have mild eczema or don't want their skin to look shiny. Examples of available gels include Doublebase® gel.

Creams

Creams are the most commonly used type of moisturiser, they are composed of an emulsion of water and oil and have a white coloured semi-solid consistency. They are popular as they are a compromise product, they rub in easier than ointments and don't leave much shine on the skin, yet they are greasier and more effective than lotions and gels. Most patients with mild and moderate eczema can control their disease with cream based moisturisers, sometimes combined with an ointment at nighttime. Cream moisturisers are not all the same and within this group you will find that some are greasier or less greasy than others. Due to this parents may find that one cream formulation moisturiser suits their child's skin better than another. Examples of available creams include

Aveeno® cream, Cetraben® cream, Diprobase® cream, E45® cream, Epaderm® cream and Oilatum® cream.

Ointments

Ointments are thick and greasy formulations of moisturiser that have a high paraffin content. The consistency is similar to petroleum jelly. They are the most effective moisturisers at hydrating the skin and are particularly useful in very dry and severe eczema. They are though more difficult to use and less cosmetically acceptable. They are difficult and rub into the skin and leave the skin looking shiny. They can cause heat trapping which can make the eczema more itchy and they can block hair follicles causing inflammation and infection. The greasiness can also stain clothing, bedding and towels. The most well known ointment moisturiser is Vaseline®. Other examples of products include Emulsifying ointment, Hydrous ointment, Diprobase® ointment, Epaderm® ointment and Hydromol® ointment.

The greasiest of all preparations is 50% liquid paraffin and 50% White Soft Parrafin, often shortened to WSP/LP 50/50, or simply 50/50. This is a useful product for patients with very severely dry eczema and I use it in children admitted to hospital but rarely give it to be used at home as it is so greasy that it is rarely tolerated. There is also a spray preparation of 50/50 called Emollin® that seems to suit some children well.

Moisturisers with additives

There are a number of moisturisers which are on the market which have additives in an attempt to make them more effective. The majority are cream formulation moisturisers which have a protein called urea added to them. Urea helps soften the keratin outer layer of the skin and assists the moisturiser in hydrating the skin itself. It is also claimed that having urea as an additive reduces itching. In very high concentrations urea containing moisturisers are used as heel balms to treat very thickened skin in this area. I have personally found these products to be of little additional value over the plain moisturisers in treating eczema, although there are a small number of children who seem to respond very well to them. Examples of products containing urea include Balneum® Plus, Calmurid®, E45® Itch Relief and Eucerin®.

There are also moisturiser preparations which have been combined with antiseptics. These are very useful products for children who get recurrent infections of their eczema. The Dermol® range includes a lotion, cream, shower emollient and bath oil. Eczmol® cream is an alternative which has a higher concentration of antiseptic. Occasionally children can become allergic to the antiseptic added to these products and they should be used on the advice of a health professional.

Using oil as a moisturiser

Since eczema was first described in Greek times it has been treated with oils. Oils are particularly useful for difficult-to-reach sites such as the scalp. For many years dermatologists have recommended olive oil, but recent studies have shown that this is not the best choice and it may make eczema worse rather than better.

Simple sunflower oil, bought from the supermarket for cooking is safe to use. Mustard oil and coconut oil are commonly used in some ethnic communities and also seem to be safe. Oils are useful as an additional therapy used alongside standard moisturisers, they should not be used as a replacement. They are not as hydrating or effective as cream and ointment formulation moisturisers. Oils are a fire risk and care should be taken.

Allergy to moisturisers

True allergy to moisturisers is exceptionally rare and I have only seen a handful of cases. The most common form allergy is an allergic contact dermatitis to additives in the moisturiser. This type of allergy is difficult to diagnose as the allergic reaction can occur up to three days after the cream has been applied. It also presents as a flare of eczema and this can be difficult to distinguish from a normal worsening of eczema. The most common additive which caused these types of allergic reactions is lanolin which is also known as wool fats. It is present in a number of moisturisers including E45®. If you suspect that your child may have this type of allergy then the correct type of allergy testing is patch testing, other types of allergy testing such as blood tests are unhelpful. Patch testing is normally undertaken by dermatologists in hospitals.

Much more commonly I am asked by parents about their child's skin goes red immediately after applying a moisturiser and whether this is an allergic reaction. When reactions occur this quickly then they are not allergic in nature and the child is not allergic to the moisturiser. In children with eczema the skin becomes very sensitive and simple mechanical action of rubbing in a cream can cause redness and inflammation. Although initially alarming this is nothing to be concerned about and it is important that you keep putting the moisturiser on. With time as the eczema is treated by the creams the skin becomes less sensitive and the redness stops.

Eczema suits

A number of companies produce special clothing for children with eczema to wear. These are often thin garments made of cotton or silk that are worn between the skin and normal clothing. The soft fabric and flat seams in this clothing reduce irritation of the skin and make children more comfortable. The clothing itself does not treat eczema although it can be used for dry wrapping as discussed below. This clothing comes in many sizes and your child will need to be measured to receive the correct sized garments. In the UK they are available on prescription through your healthcare professional.

Many parents try to incorrectly use this clothing as a barrier to prevent their children scratching. This simply does not work, children are incredibly resourceful and they will find a way through the clothing to scratch. The best way to stop children scratching is to treat the eczema, if the eczema is settled then the itching will go. Other aids to stop scratching include using mits and socks over the hands in babies and using products such as Scratchsleeves® in older children.

Wet wrapping

Both wet and dry wrapping are treatments for eczema which has not responded to standard therapies and should be initiated and supervised by a healthcare professional. This is particularly important if steroids are being used under the wrapping.

Wet wrapping is a form of bandaging used to treat children with severe eczema. It has become less popular over the past few years as it is time consuming, messy and other treatments for eczema have become available. It is though a very effective treatment, particularly at giving immediate relief a child with intractable itching. As it is difficult to do it is normally started in hospital or by a community specialist nurse. The child is first covered in moisturiser and steroid ointments, then a layer of bandages soaked in water is applied. Over this a second layer of dry bandaging is placed on top. As the first layer dries out more water can be applied and the outer layer replaced. Although the treatment is effective care must be taken not to use wet wraps if infection is present and extra care must be taken with steroid ointments as absorption of the steroid is increased under bandaging.

Dry wrapping

Dry wrapping is much simpler than wet wrapping and is particularly good for young children and babies. The child is covered in a thick layer of moisturiser, ideally an ointment, then dry bandages or a suit is placed on the child. Like with wet wrapping it must not be used if infection is suspected and care must be taken with steroid ointments. A simple and safe home technique for doing this to young babies is to cover the child in a thick layer of an ointment moisturiser then put on an old baby grow for them to sleep in. The moisturiser will soak in overnight and the baby grow will prevent stains on the bedding. In older children with eczema localised to particular areas this technique can also be used, for example using cotton gloves to treat hand eczema. The eczema suits described above can also be used to do dry wrapping.

How to Use Steroid Ointments

Key points

- Steroid ointments combined with regular moisturising are the mainstay of treating eczema
- If used correctly steroid ointments do not cause skin thinning or colour change
- The most common reason for having poorly controlled eczema is underuse of steroid ointments
- Steroids should be used regularly and not for short courses
- Always use steroid ointments, not steroid creams
- Eczema is a chronic condition and treatment needs to be continued regularly for the long term, don't stop steroids suddenly or the eczema will flare
- Do not use steroid ointments on the eyelids without specialist advice

Fears and worries surrounding steroids

Most parents I meet do not want to use steroids to treat their children's eczema. They have read on the internet and been told by health professionals that steroids are harmful and may damage their child's skin. As a parent myself I can sympathise with how difficult it is to do anything that may put your child in danger or harm them. I can though also reassure you that if you use steroid ointments properly, as described in this chapter then the chance of causing any harm to your child is infinitesimally small and in fact you are more likely to cause harm to your child by withholding such a crucial and safe treatment.

The side effects most parents are concerned about are skin thinning and colour change. These concerns go back to when steroids were first introduced fifty years ago. At the time the side effects of steroids were not fully understood and a number of people were given overly strong treatment which caused problems. Over the years fears surrounding this experience have been perpetuated and even healthcare professionals are often scared and overly cautious when using steroids ointments, particularly when prescribing for children. We have though learned huge amounts about these medications over the past decades and we can now confidently prescribe steroid ointments to children, knowing what strengths and amounts of treatment are safe to use. As I have said above significantly more harm is caused to children by under-treatment of eczema with steroid ointments rather than overtreatment.

Steroids do though have side effects and it is important to understand these when making a decision over treatment of your child. When very strong, adult strength steroids are used on children there is a risk of skin thinning, especially if used on the face. If medium strength and weak strength steroid ointments designed for children are used the chance of skin thinning is negligible. Knowing what strength of steroid to use in a particular child or on a particular location is a skill which is picked up over many years. Most healthcare professionals tend towards caution and will give weaker steroid ointments which are invariably safe. Those with significant experience such as dermatologists have the expertise and knowledge to use stronger steroid ointments.

Colour change in eczema is common and invariably due to the eczema itself rather than any treatment. Eczema related colour changes in the skin are discussed in more detail in the chapter on eczema in pigmented skin. In my career I have never seen skin colour change due to steroid ointments, even in adults who have used very strong preparations for many years. Steroids do suppress the immune system in the skin, this is how they reduce inflammation and treat eczema. This does though mean that the skin is less good at fighting infection when steroid ointments are used and the ointments should be stopped if infection is present.

If very strong steroids are used all over the body for long periods enough steroid can be absorbed into the body to develop some of the side effects seen when taking tablet steroids. Although I have occasionally seen this in adult patients I have never seen this in a child and it is not an issue of concern as long as appropriate children's strength steroid ointments are used.

How to use steroids

When steroid ointments are used there should be a gap of twenty minutes between applying the steroid and the moisturiser, if they are given too close together neither will absorb into the skin properly. There are great advocates for applying the steroid, waiting twenty minutes, then applying the moisturiser, but there are just as many advocates for doing it the other way around. In reality it probably doesn't matter in which order you apply the moisturiser and steroid, but leaving fifteen to twenty minutes to let the first treatment soak in before applying the second is important.

Unlike moisturisers that can be applied as frequently as required, steroids should be applied twice a day, in the morning and in the evening. The one exception to this is a strong steroid ointment called Elocon® which is a once daily application. Some healthcare professionals recommend increasing the frequency of applying steroids as an alternative to changing to a stronger preparation. I do not agree with this and recommend using steroid ointments a maximum of twice a day, which is the licensed regime. Steroids ointments should only be applied to areas of active eczema, patches of skin which are red, dry and inflamed. They should not be applied all over like mositurisers.

Many parents get caught in a cycle, they treat their child's eczema with a steroid until the eczema is settling, then they stop the treatment, the eczema then flares, they then go back to using the steroid. This cycle occurs as they are often given poor advice by health professionals to stop the steroid after a certain number of days and when they do this the eczema rebounds and flares. These flares can be quite severe requiring stronger steroid ointments to control them. The cycle itself can be easily broken by switching to using the steroid ointment regularly and continuously for the long term. When parents do this they find that they can drop the strength of the steroid ointment they are using, which for many is the ultimate aim.

One treatment regime is to use a weaker strength steroid continuously and alter the amount of steroid being used. The steroid is used twice a day every day and if a child's eczema is flaring then the amount of steroid ointment being used can be increased, whereas if a child's eczema is settled the amount of steroid can be reduced. Even if there is only a tiny patch of eczema it is worth treating it as you are not only treating the eczema which is visible but also preventing this patch from spreading and getting worse. The only time to stop using the steroid ointment completely is when you can see no eczema at all on the skin to treat. When this happens you should continue with moisturisers and restart the steroid ointment as soon as you see the eczema start to return.

Another treatment regime is to use a stronger steroid and alter the frequency of usage. An example would be the 'Elocon® weekender regime' where the potent steroid Elocon® is used twice weekly on a Saturday and Sunday and no steroid is used on weekdays. When a child flares the steroid can be used additionally during the week and when the eczema settles less quantity of the steroid can be used at weekends. Like with the weaker steroid regime the key is continuous usage of the steroid ointment.

When parents and patients become confident in the use of steroid ointments they can use a more advanced technique of self medicating with varying strengths of steroid. As described above the steroid is never stopped completely but the patient has two or even three strengths of steroid and varies the strength of steroid as well as the amount used depending upon the severity of the eczema. For this technique to work parents need to have had counseling by a healthcare professional so they have a good understanding of when to use the various strengths of steroid ointment.

Where to use and not use steroids

Most children with eczema are given two strengths of steroid ointment. A stronger preparation to be used on most of the skin and a weaker preparation to be used in sensitive areas. This is because the thickness of the skin varies at different body sites and in certain areas we need to be more cautious in using steroids.

On the palms, the soles and the genitals the skin is very thick and strong steroids can be used safely, even in children. On most of the rest of the body below the neck it is also safe to use stronger steroids. Sensitive areas in which we need to be more careful with steroids include the face, neck and where the skin folds in the groin and armpits. In these areas steroid ointments can be used safely, but it is better to use weaker preparations.

The only area where great caution needs to be taken is on the eyelids and skin surrounding the eyes. The skin on the eyelids is the thinnest of anywhere in the body and if steroid is absorbed into the eye this can cause serious problems. You should only ever use steroid ointments on the eyelid on the advice of a specialist dermatologist or eye specialist.

Steroid creams and ointments

The majority of steroids are available in two forms of preparation, a cream and an ointment. For example you can purchase 1% Hydrocortisone cream and 1% Hydrocortisone ointment. This is similar to moisturisers that can be either light creams or greasy ointments. Cream based steroids are white in colour and are easy to rub in without leaving a sheen on the skin. Ointment based steroids are greasy, more difficult to rub in and leave the skin looking shiny. Children and parents often prefer to use the cream preparation steroids as they are easier to rub in and more cosmetically acceptable. Some healthcare professionals also tend to prescribe the cream preparations as they are mostly cheaper. In fact nearly every child with eczema should be using steroid ointments, not creams.

As steroid ointments have a greasy base they moisturise the skin at the same time as delivering the steroid, this is important as eczema is a dry skin condition. Steroid creams on the other hand can actually dry the skin out and the cream base can negate many of the benefits of the steroid itself. Steroid creams also have a shorter shelf life and because of this they contain additional chemicals and preservatives. Steroid ointments have a natural long shelf life and do not require these chemicals giving a simpler preparation that children are less likely to react to. Steroid ointments are more effective and in the long run you need to use less of them. It is exceptionally rare for me to prescribe a steroid cream and nearly all children with eczema should be treated with steroid ointments. Switching from a steroid cream to a steroid ointment of the same strength can make a huge difference and lead to much better control of a child's eczema.

Types of Steroid Ointment

Key points

- There are a large number of steroids on the market
- It is important to understand the different strengths of steroid and when they should be used
- Some steroids preparations are mixed with antibiotics and antifungal medications
- The finger-tip-unit is a way the measure the amount of steroid to use
- There are newer alternatives to steroid ointments and there are advantages and disadvantages to using these products

Types of steroid available

There are a huge number of different steroid ointments on the market and it is difficult and confusing to understand the differences between them. To make this easier doctors classify steroids into four groups depending on how strong they are, these groups are mild, moderate, potent and super potent. This is though just a guide and there are differences in the strength of steroids even within the same group.

To add to the difficulty most steroid ointments also have two names, a brand name and a name for the actual steroid used in the ointment. For example Betnovate® is the brand name for a potent steroid produced by the pharmaceutical company Glaxosmithkline. The active ingredient in Betnovate® is 0.1% betamethasone valerate which is the actual steroid. Glaxosmithkline are not the only company to produce a steroid ointment with this particular steroid and your doctor may prescribe a generic 0.1% betamethasone valerate produced by a different company.

Some steroid ointments have the same name and come in different strengths. For example there is a steroid ointment called Synalar® which is potent in strength, Synalar 1 in 4 dilution® which is moderate in strength and Synalar 1 in 10 dilution® which is mild in strength.

Steroid combination products

Steroid ointments are available that are mixed together with antibiotics, antifungal medications and antiseptics. This does seem like a great idea as a steroid combined with an antibiotic would treat both the eczema and any bacterial infection on the skin. In reality there are disadvantages to using these products and they should be used with caution.

Children with eczema are sensitive to chemicals and may develop an allergy to the antibiotics and other drugs added to the products. There is also now significant bacterial resistance to some of the antibiotics used in these products as they have been overused. Lastly many of these combination products are only available as a cream preparation and you lose the benefits of using steroid ointments.

Mild steroids

Mild strength steroids are the weakest available, this has the advantage of them being very safe, but they are also not that effective at treating eczema. For most young children who have mild eczema then this may be the only strength of steroid they need. In general it is safe to use this strength of steroid on the body of all children, even newborn babies. Some caution needs to be used when using even mild steroids on the face and you should consultant with a healthcare professional before doing this. As with all steroids they should not be used on the eyelids unless your child is under the care of a specialist. In the UK 1% hydrocortisone is available to buy over the counter at chemists without the need for a prescription; it is restricted for use in children over ten years of age for a maximum of one week of usage.

Hydrocortisone is the most well known and commonly used mild steroid. It is available as a cream and an ointment and comes in various strengths. 1% Hydrocortisone is the standard strength and the only strength I recommend using. Lower strengths are available at 0.5% and 0.1% (Dioderm®) but I have found these to be ineffective. A stronger 2.5% strength is also available but again I do not recommend using this, if 1% Hydrocortisone is ineffective then it is best to step up to a moderate strength steroid. Synalar 1 in 10® is an alternative to hydrocortisone, although this is only available as a cream preparation. For the vast majority of patients I would recommend they use 1% Hydrocortisone ointment as the mild strength steroid of choice to treat eczema.

Canesten® HC and Daktacort® are combination preparations of 1% Hydrocortisone mixed with antifungal medications. These can be useful products when treating seborrhoeic dermatitis but otherwise have limited use in treating eczema. Fucidin® H is a combination of 1% Hydrocortisone with an antibiotic. In some areas the bacteria which tend to infect eczema are resistant to the antibiotic contained in Fucidin® H and because of this I rarely use the product. Timodine® is combination of 0.5% hydrocortisone with an antiseptic and antifungal. This can be useful in recurrently infected mild eczema.

Moderate steroids

Moderate strength steroids are the mainstay of treatment for children with moderate and severe eczema. In toddlers and older children it is safe to use moderate strength steroids on the body. They should only be used on the face or other sensitive sites on the advice of a specialist. They should also only be used in children under one year of age on the advice of a specialist.

Betnovate-RD®, Eumovate®, Modrasone® and Synalar® 1 in 4 are all moderate strength steroids that are available in cream and ointment preparations. Eumovate® tends to be the most commonly used steroid ointment in this group. Although still moderate in strength Betnovate-RD® is considered to be slightly stronger than the others in this group. I tend to use Eumovate® ointment as my steroid of choice for moderate eczema, stepping up to Betnovate-RD® if I need something a little stronger. There is though little to choose between the steroids in this group.

Trimovate® is a combination product which combines the steroid used in Eumovate® with an antibiotic and antifungal medication. Trimovate® is only available as a cream preparation; it is yellow in colour and can stain clothing. Like other combination products children can become allergic to the components of this cream and it should only be used on specialist advice.

Potent steroids

Potent steroids are designed for adults and adult skin. They are strong medications that can cause skin thinning and other problems when used inappropriately in children. Potent steroids should never be used on the face or on other sensitive sites. They are only used in children with severe eczema, for limited periods of time and under the supervision of a dermatologist.

Betnovate®, Elocon®, Cutivate®, Diprosone®, Locoid®, Metosyn® and Synalar® are all potent steroids and need to be used with great care in children. Betnovate-C®, Betnovate-N®, Fucibet®, Synalar-C® and Synalar-N® are all combination products with potent steroids and antibiotics mixed together. Lotriderm® is a potent steroid mixed with an antifungal medication.

Super potent steroids

Super potent strength steroids are only used in children in the most exceptional of circumstances. When steroids of this strength are used it must be under the close supervision of a consultant dermatologist. These creams should never be prescribed by family doctors or nurse specialists for use in children. Dermovate® and Nerisone Forte® are both super potent strength steroids. If you are ever prescribed these medications by anyone other than a consultant dermatologist then do not use them and seek a second opinion.

Amounts of steroid to use

It can be difficult to gauge how much steroid to use; one method is to use a guide known as a finger tip unit. If you squeeze out a length of cream from the end of your fingertip to the first joint this is one finger tip unit. One finger tip unit weights about half a gram and can be used to cover an area the size of two palm prints of skin. Although fairly accurate using finger tip units is fiddly and it can be difficult to keep track.

As an alternative guide I have found parents find it easier to judge how long a tube of steroid ointment should last them. I always recommend that children are prescribed the larger 100g tubes of steroid ointment. One of these large tubes should last about 2 months for a baby, 6 weeks for a toddler and 1 month for a school age child. It is of course dependant on how large the child is, how strong the steroid ointment is and how much of their skin is affects by eczema. If though you aim to use these quantities then you should be getting good treatment of the eczema without causing side effects.

Other Steroid Preparations

As well as creams and ointments steroids are available in other preparations for treating eczema in difficult sites. Haelan® tape is a sticky tape impregnated with a moderate strength steroid. It is particularly useful for treating cracked fingertips and small localised areas of eczema. The tape is usually applied for 12 hours and then removed. In children it is often easiest to apply it overnight and take it off in the morning.

Steroids are also available in lotions, gels and foams to be used in hairy areas such as the scalp. In most cases of eczema the scalp can be treated with moisturisers alone, but in some children steroids are required. As there are no mild or moderate strength steroid scalp applications in production we have to use adult potent strength steroids. When this is required I normally advise parents to use the product two or three times a week, rather than every day, and when the eczema is controlled to try and reduce the frequency of application to once weekly.

Prednisolone is a tablet steroid that is very occasionally given to treat severe flares of eczema. Although safe in short courses it is dangerous to stay on steroid tablets for long periods. If a child has such severe eczema that they require courses of tablet steroids then they should be under the care of a dermatologist.

Alternatives to steroids

In the past few years new products have been developed as alternatives to topical steroids. These products are known as immune modulators and do not cause skin thinning. They are cream preparations of tablets which doctors have used for many years to suppress the immune system in patients who have undergone an organ transplant. They should be used in children who have failed treatment with steroids or who cannot use steroids. These creams should only be prescribed by doctors with experience in using them.

Elidel® is a cream that contains the active ingredient Pimecrolimus. It is licensed to be used in children over the age of two years twice daily for the short term and intermittently in the long term. I have found its strength to be similar to mild steroid ointments.

Protopic® is an ointment that contains the active ingredient tacrolimus. It comes in two strengths, the 0.03% should be used in children between two and sixteen years of age and the 0.1% should be used in adults and children over sixteen years of age. Both ointments should be used twice daily for two weeks, then reduced to once daily then used intermittently in the long term. I have this preparation to be more effective but less cosmetically acceptable than Elidel®.

In my experience these products are very useful when used, but only in certain, selected children. The creams are particularly good at treating eczema around the eyes where we do not like using steroids. The main problem with using these creams is that they cause stinging when they are applied to the skin. The stinging lasts fifteen to twenty minutes then subsides, with repeated use stinging becomes less of a problem. Like with steroids it is important to stop the creams if there is any infection as they do impair the skins ability to fight infections.

Treatments for Less Common Types of Eczema

Key points

- There are many less common subtypes of eczema
- These types of eczema often require different treatments to standard eczema

Seborrhoeic Dermatitis

Seborrhoeic dermatitis is a form of eczema that tends to affect young babies and teenagers. The eczema is greasy, scaly and affects the face and trunk. It is often associated with cradle cap in young children and dandruff in adults. Moisturisers are less important in this type of eczema although they are useful in softening the scale. As this condition is partly due to an overgrowth of yeast on the skin antifungal treatments are often used. Ketoconazole shampoo is an antifungal shampoo that can be both on the scalp and also on the body as a shower gel. Steroid ointments either as a single agent or combined with antifungals in products such as Daktacort® are often effective. Coal tar based products, which are normally used in psoriasis can be used in resistant cases.

Cradle Cap

Many children have cradle cap as young babies, it presents as thick greasy scales on the scalp. In most cases medications are not needed. Sunflower oil can be used to soften the scales and they can be removed gently with a comb. Some mothers find it relaxing to pick the scales off whilst breastfeeding, which is perfectly safe, if a little messy. For more severe cases medicated shampoos can be used and left on the scalp for five to ten minutes before removing. Options include anti-dandruff shampoos such as Head and Shoulders®, coal tar shampoos such as T-gel® and the antifungal shampoo Nizoral®. In resistant cases it is often useful to alternate two or three of the shampoos listed above. It is rare that steroid scalp applications are required for this condition.

Nappy Rash

All babies develop nappy rash regardless of how diligently parents change the child's nappies. It is caused by the nappy contents pressing against the skin leading to irritation, inflammation and eczema. The most important thing in treating nappy rash is to change the nappy frequently, especially after the baby has been to the toilet. Some healthcare professionals advocate leaving the nappy off for long periods to 'air' the area. Personally I don't find this particularly effective and it both impractical and potentially very messy.

Barrier creams are very useful, as the name implies they act as a barrier protecting the skin from the nappy contents. In general the thicker the barrier cream the better, with my children I have found Metanium® to be more effective than Sudocrem®. A thick layer of the cream should be applied around the bottom, genitals and groin folds at every nappy change. In girls it is important to apply the cream from front-to-back to protect the genitals from bacteria which live around the bottom. Greasy ointments such as '50/50' can be used as an alternative but be aware that they can impair the absorption in disposable nappies.

Steroids should be used with great care in nappy rash and only on the advice of a healthcare professional. Infection, particularly with the yeast candida, can mimic nappy rash and steroids will make this worse rather than better. If your child has severe nappy rash and it is not responding to standard treatment then it is important to consultant your doctor to rule out other, rare rashes that can occur in this area.

Lip Licking Dermatitis

Commonly seen in toddlers, eczema develops around the mouth due to repetitive licking. Licking the eczema gives a feeling of temporary relief but also exacerbates the problem leading to a cycle of worsening eczema and increased licking. If the cycle can be broken then rash resolves completely and often does not reoccur. The key to breaking the cycle is applying a greasy ointment moisturiser around the mouth twenty or thirty times a day for a few weeks. The moisturiser acts a barrier protecting the skin as well treating the eczema. It is also non-toxic and tastes foul, discouraging the child from licking the area. If this method does not work then you should seek medical advice to confirm the diagnosis. I find steroid creams are rarely needed for this condition and it is better to avoid using them if possible.

Discoid Eczema

In discoid eczema children have round patches of thickened eczema on the arms, legs and trunk. As the eczema is often thickened stronger steroid ointments can be applied including using potent strength steroids for short periods on the advice of healthcare professionals. There is also an infective component to this type of eczema and some dermatologists recommend using combination steroid prodcuts that include an antibiotic. Personally I find the Dermol® 600 antiseptic bath oil useful in this type of eczema when used alongside a regular steroid ointment and moisturiser.

Pompholyx Eczema

In pompholyx eczema children develop thousands of tiny blisters on the hands and feet, these then dry up leading to painful cracks in the skin. When in the blister stage steroid creams rather than ointments should be used as they help dry up the blisters. Often strong potent strength steroids are required. It is safe use potent steroids on the hands and feet in children for short periods, although this should be supervised by a healthcare professional. If the blisters become very big they can be burst with a sterile needle.

As the eczema moves into the dry, cracked phase treatment is switched to greasy ointment moisturiser and a steroid ointment. With any hand eczema it is important to avoid soaps and wash the hands with a soap substitute. Haelan® tape is particularly useful for cracks of eczema on the fingers. For very deep cracks that do not heal Super Glue® can be used to stick the edges of the skin together and form a protective barrier.

Juvenile Plantar Dermatosis

Most commonly seen in school aged boys they get shiny, cracked eczema on the soles of feet, particularly on the forefoot. It is more common in children with other types of eczema and is due to friction between the foot and synthetic materials found in socks and shoes. It is often mistaken for fungal infection. Unlike other types of eczema there is very little role for steroid creams. It is though important that the skin is well moisturised with a greasy ointment. Children should be encouraged to 'air' the feet as much as possible, walking around in bare feet when at home. When going out they should wear two layers of cotton socks and a pair of well fitting leather shoes. Simple plasters and bandaging will speed up the healing of fissures caused by the condition.

Hand Dermatitis

Hand dermatitis is a chronic eczema of the hands leading to permanently dry, inflamed skin and deep cracks and fissures. It is treatable but requires a huge and sustained effort from the patient. A greasy ointment based moisturiser should be applied to hands ten to twenty times a day. It is vital to avoid hand contact with any irritants such as soap, cleaning products and washing up liquid. Hands should be washed with a moisturiser used as a soap substitute rather than with soap. After washing the moisturiser should be applied again. Overnight patients should let a thick layer of moisturiser soak in under white cotton gloves. Often potent strength steroids ointments are required to treat this condition but they should only be used on the advice of a healthcare professional. It is very common for this type of eczema to become chronic and an aggressive treatment regime needs to be kept up for many years to return the skin back to normal.

Bath Time

Key points

- Bath time should be a fun and enjoyable experience
- Bathing sooths eczema and gives temporary relief from itching
- If done properly bathing and showering can be beneficial to treating eczema
- Soaps, bubble baths, shower gels and shampoos must all be avoided
- Bath oils and soap substitutes should be used for cleaning
- A good layer of moisturiser should be applied after bathing

How often?

There are few things in eczema health professionals argue about more than frequency of bathing in eczema. Some feel that bathing is always bad for eczema and should be done as infrequently as twice a week. Others feel it is a very good way to treat eczema and children should be bathed up to three times a day. My view is that as long as bathing is done correctly it is good for eczema, but it should it should not be overdone. If done properly bathing is time consuming and for practical reasons bathing once a day, prior to going to bed seems to be the best compromise.

What to avoid?

Soaps should be avoided as they have an irritant and drying effect on eczema. Children should be cleaned with the bath water and a soap substitute. Unfortunately many cosmetic companies produce soap based products that claim to be gentle on the skin, pH neutral, fragrance free and child friendly. Despite these claims they are not good for eczema and should all be avoided. This advice also applies to bubble baths, shampoos, conditioners and shower gels. Children only start to produce oil on their hair in sufficient quantities to look greasy when they start puberty. Before then shampoos and conditioners are simply not needed.

Hair can be washed in the bath water mixed with a bath oil, this is all that is required. My children have never used shampoo and their hair is as clean and healthy looking as any of their friends. In older children where shampoo is required, they should use the smallest possible quantities and wash it out quickly. This should be done at the end of bath time so they are not sitting in the shampoo suds for a long time. I cannot overemphasise how bad soaps are for eczema and how many parents fall into the mistake of using soaps marketed as sensitive or child friendly.

Soap substitutes

Soap substitutes are moisturisers that can be used to clean the skin instead of soaps. It is important to avoid soaps as they dry the skin and flare eczema. Nearly all moisturisers can also be used as soap substitutes although many people find lotions to be the easiest to use.

When washing your hands a small amount of the moisturiser should be placed in the palm and then spread to give the hands a light coating. Instead of rubbing this in, the hands should then be placed in water and rubbed together, a lather will then form which is rinsed off. Following washing a second layer of moisturiser should be rubbed into the skin in the normal manner. For baths and showers it is often easiest to apply a thin layer of the moisturiser before getting in, then rubbing into a lather once in the water. If doing this your child will be very slippery and care needs to be taken. Even when using a soap substitute it remains important to apply a second layer of moisturiser after drying.

Bath oils

Bath oils are liquid oils that are poured into a bath and dissolve, sometimes giving a white cloudy appearance to the bath. They are meant to be diluted and not applied onto the skin as a 'leave on' product. Using a bath oil prevents the skin drying out during bath time and gives a moisturising effect. In general one capful is used in a baby bath and two capfuls are used in a full sized bath. It is important to mix the bath around to make sure the oil is well dispersed. Many of the bath oils are from the same range as moisturisers and have the same brand name. For example the Oilatum® range includes two bath oils and a moisturiser.

There is little to choose between different bath oils although parents will notice that some mix in better with the water than others leaving less residue. I personally have found the Hydromol® bath and shower emollient the most cosmetically acceptable of the brands I have tried. Other commonly used bath oils include Aveeno® bath oil, Balneum® bath oil, Cetraben® emollient bath additive, Dermalo® bath emollient, Diprobath®, Doublebase® emollient bath additive, E45® Emollient bath oil, Oilatum® emollient bath additive and Oilatum® junior emollient bath additive.

Parents should be aware of what ingredients are used in bath oils as rarely children can be allergic to some of these compounds. An example I saw was a young boy who reacted to Aveeno® bath oil which contains oatmeal, he was later shown to have allergy to oats. Lanolin which is also known as wool alcohols is present in Dermalo® bath emollient and both Oilatum® bath oils. Balneum® bath oil contains soya oil. Fragrances are found in Aveeno® bath oil, Balneum® bath oil and both Oilatum® bath oils.

Balneum Plus® bath oil contains lauromacrogols, chemicals which have local anaesthetic properties. Manufacturers claim that lauromacrogols have soothing properties for eczema. Personally I have never seen any dramatic differences between standard products and those which contain this additional ingredient, but I keep an open mind.

Dermol® 600 bath emollient and Oilatum® Plus bath additive are bath oils that contain antiseptics. They are useful particularly in children who get recurrent infections of their eczema. Parents should though consider that any chemical they put on their child's skin has the potential to cause an allergic reaction and many dermatologists advocate 'keeping it simple' and using products with the least amount of ingredients as possible.

How to bathe children with eczema

Children should be bathed in a luke warm bath and you should always use a bath thermometer to check it is not too hot. Bath oil should be poured into the bath and mixed in well. The bath and child are going to be very slippery and always use a shower mat for extra grip in full sized baths. Keep the bath between one quarter and one third full but no more in case the child falls over. Before putting the child in the bath cover them in a layer of your soap substitute. Once in the bath use the water to lather up the soap substitute and clean the child. Then spend a good ten minutes playing, bath time is supposed to be fun! At the end of the bath carefully transfer the child onto a toweling mat and pat them dry with a cotton towel. Once dry apply a good layer of moisturiser and dress.

Many parents are concerned as their child becomes very red at bath time and the eczema often looks angry. This is nothing to be concerned about. As a normal response to being warm in the bath the blood vessels in the skin dilate making the skin turn red. With this the eczema often does look angrier for a short time and this is sometimes made worse by the physical drying and rubbing of creams into the skin. Although worrying at the time, this is only temporary and overall the child will benefit from a properly undertaken bath.

Showering

Some children do not have access to a bath or simply prefer showering. Children with eczema do not need to have baths and it is quite reasonable for them to have showers as an alternative. Like with baths a once a day shower is appropriate. You should avoid shampoos, soaps and shower gels all of which will flare eczema. A soap substitute should be used for cleaning in the shower and a number of companies produce moisturisers in shower gel like containers for this purpose. Examples include Doublebase® emollient shower gel, Oilatum®shower emollient, Dermol® 200 shower emollient and E45® shower emollient cream. After the shower the child should be gently patted dry and then a good layer of moisturiser should be applied just like after having a bath.

Swimming

Most parents find that swimming flares their child's eczema. This is due to the chlorine in the swimming pool which is an irritant. Saying this most children love swimming and if at all possible children with eczema should be allowed to enjoy this healthy activity. To protect your child a thick layer of a greasy ointment moisturiser should be applied before swimming, 50/50 WSP/LP is particularly good for this. After swimming your child should be well washed under the shower whilst using a soap substitute. Lastly, another layer of moisturiser should be applied. Most parents find that as long as they are sensible and follow the guidance above then their children can swim happily. There are though a small number of children with severe eczema who cannot tolerate swimming.

Sleeping

Key points

- Poor sleeping is one of the most difficult and stressful aspects of looking after a child with eczema

- Eczema is always more itchy at nighttime

- Most children with bad eczema have trouble sleeping

- Treating eczema well during the day is the key to helping children sleep at night

- Keep children cool, with short nails and sleeping in their own bed

- Anti-histamines should only be used for short periods when the eczema flares and are best given at night

- Do not wake your child up to apply creams overnight.

Getting a good night's sleep

One thing nearly all parents tell me is how their child's eczema is worse at bed time. Time and again I hear stories of children being up all night scratching and parents diligently sitting by their beds trying the stop them. The child becomes sleep deprived and irritable, the parents become sleep deprived and irritable. It is an ever worsening cycle which is making everyone miserable and unhappy.

There are a few reasons why eczema is worse at night. Mostly it is due to heat, at night children are snuggled under duvets and blankets and get really quite warm. The heat does not flare the eczema, but it does make it itchier and children scratch. Another reason is distraction, during the day children busy doing things and concentration is taken away from scratching, but at night there is little else to occupy them and they concentrate on the itching. Some children also get what doctors call secondary gain from this. They realize that if they scratch then they get attention from their parents and their parents will stay in their room with them. Because they like having this attention they will scratch more to get more of what they want.

The best way to get round this problem is to treat the eczema. If the eczema is well treated with moisturisers and steroids then it will not itch, it will not be worse at night and they will sleep better. As they sleep better they will be happier, their stress hormones will be reduced and the eczema will improve. It is this 'getting better' cycle that you want, not the ever worsening cycle described above.

It is also important to keep the child cool to prevent the heat related flare of itching. Use light, cotton bed clothing, a summer duvet, fewer blankets, turn the heating down, even keep the window open. It is a balance, you do not want your child to be cold, but nor should they be hot. Keeping fingernails cut short and filed blunt will also help, making the fingers less effective implements for scratching.

Lastly you should try and resist letting your child sleep in your bed. It is so tempting to have them in easy reach, to comfort them and physically stop them scratching. It does though make things worse as they will get very warm sleeping next to you. It is also not recommended to sleep in the bed as your child due to the increased risk of cot death. Perhaps more importantly it is not good for your sleep nor for your relationship with your partner. You need a good night's sleep so you are well rested and happy and can do the best for your child.

Anti-histamines

Anti-histamines are tablets or syrups that some doctors prescribe to help with itching and sleeping. Histamine is a chemical produced by the body as part of the allergy pathway and leads to inflammation and itching. Anti-histamine tablets block the histamine chemical thereby reducing inflammation and itch. As a side effect most anti-histamines are also sedating and make children sleepy. There are two types of anti-histamine medications – sedating and non-sedating. In reality even non-sedating anti-histamines cause some drowsiness. Anti-histamines are extremely safe medicines and can be given to even very young children if prescribed in the correct dose.

In eczema they tend to be useful when given for short periods, particularly at night when they will both reduced itch and help sleep. I do not find them useful during the day as such high doses are required to stop children itching that they become very sleepy and sedated. If your child is very itchy it is normally a sign that the eczema is under-treated and the best way to stop them itching is to increase the amounts of steroid and moisturiser that you are using. The itching of eczema does not involve histamine and as such anti-histamines are not great at reducing itch unless there is also urticaria.

Children also rapidly become resistant to anti-histamines and you will find after a few weeks of regular use they simply no longer work. I do not prescribe anti-histamines to be used regularly for this reason. They are though very useful medicines when used for a few days at time when a child's eczema has flared and they are having trouble sleeping.

Commonly used antihistamines include Piriton® (Chlorphenamine maleate), Cetirizine, Neoclarityn® (Desloratidine), Loratidine, Vallergan® (Alimemazine tartrate) and Ucerax® (Hydroxyzine hydrochloride).

Treating eczema at night

I have spoken to parents who wake their children up at night to apply layers of moisturiser. Although they are trying to do the best for their child, this is best not done. If the eczema is treated properly it simply is not necessary and it is important for the child to have a good unbroken night's sleep.

If your child has very dry skin which needs regular moisturising the best treatment overnight is dry wrapping with a greasy ointment as described earlier. With proper preparation before bedtime your child can both have a good night's sleep and have good treatment for their eczema.

Flares

Key points

- As part of the natural process of eczema the disease flares and settles
- Rarely if ever can a cause be found for particular flares
- Few flares are due to allergic reactions to foods
- Flares are best prevented by treating the underlying eczema
- Flares are best treated by increasing the amount or strength of steroid ointment being used

Flares of eczema

Eczema is a condition that goes through cycles of flaring and settling. It is common for a child's eczema to be well controlled for weeks or even months and then deteriorate and get worse, often for no reason that can be identified. The eczema can get worse over hours, days or weeks and remain bad for days or even weeks. Flares of eczema are very upsetting for parents. They are often doing everything right, putting all the creams on but their child still flares. Some parents can be driven to become desperate beyond reason to find out why their child's eczema is flaring and how they can stop it.

Inflammatory flares of eczema

The vast majority of flares are due to no reason at all. It is very hard for parents to accept this but eczema is a condition that cycles. As part of the natural cycle of eczema it goes through phases where it gets worse and gets better. I like to think of these as inflammatory flares of eczema as they are caused by increased inflammation of the skin rather than any infection or allergy. There is nothing a parent can do to completely

52

prevent inflammatory flares of eczema, although they can though reduce the likelihood of flares and treat flares effectively when they do occur.

Other causes of flares

Most parents are led astray by the internet and even healthcare professionals into thinking that allergic reactions to foods cause eczema to flare. In fact very few flares of eczema are caused by allergic reactions to food as discussed in the chapter on allergy. Infection is a potentially more serious cause of eczema flaring. It is important that you recognise when our child's eczema is infected so they can receive the correct treatment. This is discussed in more detail in the chapter on infection.

Most patients with eczema find it is worse during the winter months. There are likely to be a number of reasons for this including lack of sunshine, dampness, cold and changes in humidity. Some people find that certain types of clothing can make eczema worse and advocate only wearing cotton clothing. I am not particularly convinced by the need to only wear cotton clothing and I find it is more important to keep a child in clothes they feel comfortable in regardless of what the garment is made from.

Stress is a well known cause of eczema flares. I often see patients whose eczema has flared after bereavement or other stressful event. It is also common to see children's eczema worsen around school examinations. Sometimes a cycle can develop where patients get stressed because of their eczema, this makes the eczema worse and then they stress more due to the worse eczema. Often a short course of strong steroid ointments is required to break this cycle.

How hormones affect eczema is very complicated and not fully understood. It is though known that some women and girls eczema flares at the time of having their period. Pregnancy tends to settle eczema in most patients, although in some cases it can make it worse.

What does not cause flares

It was previous thought that hard water may worsen eczema and many websites claim that water softening devices will lead to a miraculous improvement of your child's eczema. In fact a large study published in 2011 showed clearly that installing a water softening devices did not affect children's eczema.

Many people also believe that washing powders and fabric conditioners cause flares of eczema. There has been a study looking at biological and non-biological washing powders and no difference was found. I would though recommend that clothes are well rinsed after washing and softeners are avoided. Probiotics have also been shown to have no benefit in eczema, neither is there any research evidence that wearing cotton clothing is beneficial. It does though make sense to wear comfortable, loose clothes and to wash new clothes before wearing them to remove any chemical residues.

How to reduce the likelihood of flares

The best way to reduce the likelihood of eczema flaring is to treat the skin well. Skin which is well moisturised and kept away from irritants like soap is less likely to flare. This is why it is so important to moisturise all of the skin and not just the areas with eczema. When the eczema itself is well treated with a regular steroid it is less likely to flare.

The most common reason for eczema to flare is under-treatment of existing eczema and this is why I always advise that parents should use the steroids and moisturisers regularly every day rather than stopping and starting them. Flares can also be precipitated by irritants and even a single lapse by allowing your child to use a bubble bath or putting soap on their skin can set off a flare. This is why it is so hard to have a child with eczema and why the treatment can be so demanding.

How to treat flares of eczema

The key to treating flares of eczema is to treat them early. As soon as you see new patches of eczema or a worsening of eczema you should treat it aggressively to stop the flare before it has chance to become established. This is one of the commonest things I speak to parents about, often parents wait for the eczema to become an established flare before increasing treatment, rather than doing this as soon as it appears. If you treat a small patch of new eczema with steroid it will prevent it become a large patch that is more difficult to treat. When treating a flare of eczema there are two approaches, one approach it to use larger quantities of steroids, the other is to switch to a stronger preparation of steroid. Your healthcare professional should have discussed this with you and put in place a plan for what you are supposed to do when the eczema flares.

If scratching is major problem then a short course of antihistamines can be useful whilst waiting for the steroid treatment to work. It is also worthwhile keeping your child's nails short and blunt by cutting and filing them every day.

Alternative Therapies

Key points

- Alternative therapies can be used to complement standard medical treatment, not replace them

- Hypnosis, psychological therapies and acupuncture can reduce stress levels which can help eczema

- Nearly all children receive adequate vitamins and minerals with their normal diet and do not benefit from supplements

- Beware miracle cures and herbal creams which may contain harmful chemicals

Should I use alternative therapies?

The treatment of eczema is difficult, time consuming and when done wrong ineffective. Parents may look to alternative or complementary therapies if medical therapies are not working, or if they are scared of applying medications to their child's skin. When used properly alternative therapies can be effective, particularly therapies which reduce stress, one of the causes of eczema flares. Alternative therapies should though only be used as an adjunct to standard treatment, not a replacement. Unfortunately I have seen a number of children hospitalised with severe flares of eczema after stopping their medical treatments when starting an alternative therapy. Studies have shown that about half of people with eczema have tried alternative therapies and most got no benefit or their eczema got worse.

Parents should also beware and realize that the alternative therapy market is not regulated, alternative practitioners are not trained doctors and they are not insured or qualified to make medical diagnoses or initiate medical treatments. There are also a small number of alternative practitioners who take financial advantage of desperate parents with extravagant and untruthful claims over the effectiveness of their treatments.

Natural Moisturisers

In the chapter on moisturisers I have discussed how oils such as sunflower oil and coconut oil can be used as moisturisers. Although effective, particularly for the scalp they are not as greasy as ointment based moisturisers and children with very dry skin may find them ineffective. A number of the more commercial preparations such as cocoa butter and sweet almond oil contain added preservatives and fragrances that your child may react to. Always read the ingredients carefully and try to use moisturisers with as few ingredients as possible. This same advice applies to preparations containing aloe vera and tea tree oil. Although it is thought that tea tree oil has some antiseptic properties it is toxic when ingested and can cause skin irritation in some children.

Dietary supplements

Lack of certain vitamins and minerals can flare eczema, but there is no evidence that dietary supplements improve eczema in most children. Every child with eczema should have a balanced diet with plenty of fruit and vegetables. Like with any child, treats are allowed, but always in moderation. Taking a daily child's multivitamin tablet is unlikely to help eczema, but nor will it cause any harm. Beware super high dose preparations of vitamins which can be dangerous. There is a lot of research currently being undertaken into the effects of vitamin D on eczema and if you are concerned that your child may have vitamin D deficiency your doctor can test this with a simple blood test. If your child has proven vitamin D deficiency then replacing this may help their eczema. If your child has normal vitamin D levels then extra amounts of the vitamin are unlikely to help and may be harmful.

Hypnosis and psychological therapies

A study looking at adults and children with severe, treatment resistant eczema did find benefit after they had undergone hypnotherapy. Although not working directly on the eczema, hypnotherapy will reduce stress, help sleep and can help the repetitive psychological dependency on scratching. Other psychological therapies may also help certain, selected people with eczema. Like with all alternative therapies these are an adjunct to be used alongside standard medical treatments.

Acupuncture

There is very little good research looking at how effective acupuncture is in eczema. It has though been shown to reduce stress which can be helpful. It is highly unlikely to cause any harm. Given the nature of acupuncture it is probably best not to be used in young children.

Chinese herbal products

It is very hard to know if Chinese herbal products help eczema. There are though concerns over the purity of different herbal concoctions. There have been cases of herbal preparations being toxic, interacting with medications and containing strong steroids. For these reasons I advise against the use of these products.

Evening primrose oil

Evening primrose oil has been used both as a supplement by mouth and applied directly onto the skin to treat eczema. It is thought to have anti-inflammatory properties and for a time was thought to improve eczema. More recent larger studies have shown that evening primrose oil by mouth does not help eczema. It also interacts with certain important medicines and if taken for prolonged periods can cause serious harm. For these reasons I advise against the use of this product.

Steroids in Herbal Creams

There have been a number of high profile cases of children being harmed by applying herbal creams that contained very strong adult strength steroids. In all the cases the creams claimed to be natural and herbal and did not mention on the packaging that they contained steroids. In most cases the creams were imported from Africa and South Asia. Recently both Wau Wa cream and Muijiza cream were available to buy on a well known commercial website with no warning that they contained adult strength steroids. In another example of eleven Chinese herbal remedies obtained in London eight contained high strength steroids. Similarly in Birmingham twenty of twenty four herbal creams analysed contained steroids.

Using herbal creams containing adult strength steroids on a child can lead to serious harm to your child. Always obtain your creams from a reputable supplier and if you are unsure check with your healthcare professional before using them. If you are concerned that a cream may contain steroid then contact the Medicine and Healthcare Products Regulatory Agency (MHRA).

Infection and Eczema

Key points

- Eczema is most commonly infected by bacteria which make it go weepy and crusty
- When eczema gets infected steroid treatment should be stopped and tablet/syrup antibiotics should be used for treatment
- Cream based antibiotics are not very helpful and in general should be avoided
- Moisturisers and bath oils containing antiseptics can be useful to prevent recurrent infected episodes
- Eczema herpeticum is a rare but serious viral infection of eczema and immediate medical help should be sought.

Bacterial infections

Most eczema infections are due to bacteria. The actual bacteria which cause infections are very common bugs that live on all of our skins. In children with eczema there are more of the bacteria and when they spread into breaks in the skin they cause infection. A simple way to tell if eczema is infected is to see if it is wet or dry. Normally eczema is a dry skin condition, but when infected it becomes weepy and wet. It may also become crusty, especially if the crust has a golden colour to it. When eczema is infected steroid treatments will not work and if your child develops some eczema that does not respond to steroid treatment then you should consider infection and seek help from a healthcare professional.

How to prevent infections

The best way to stop eczema getting infected is to treat it well with steroids and moisturisers. If the eczema is well treated then there will be fewer breaks in the skin for bacteria to infect. Despite good treatment there are though a small group of children who get repetitive infections one after another. It is a difficult situation as most anti-bacterial soaps are very harsh and will flare eczema making it worse. For these patients the moisturisers and bath oils that contain antiseptics such as the Dermol® range are a very useful way to reduce the amount of bacteria on the skin and reduce infections. These products are discussed in more detail in the chapter on moisturisers. In addition the inside of the nose is a place which tends to harbor bacteria and sometimes doctors will take swabs from the nose and treat inside the nose with cream based antibiotics. Lastly, it is important to recognise bacterial infection early and seek treatment before it spreads. Very rarely infection can spread from the skin into the blood and this can be very serious.

Bleach Baths

Bleach baths are a method of reducing the amount of bacteria on the skin of children with eczema. There is some research evidence that they can reduce episodes of infection in children who present with recurrent eczema infections. One quarter of a cup of thin bleach should be mixed well into a full bathtub of water and the child should bathe for five to ten minutes before rinsing with plain water. The head should not be submerged and bleach baths should not be used more than twice a week.

I do not recommend the use of bleach baths, I do believe that they work, but the potential dangers are great. In my experience as a parent it is best to keep bleach well out of reach of children. Vinegar baths are another alternative where one cup of vinegar is added to the bath giving an antiseptic effect. Although there are no comparison studies I believe bath oils containing antiseptics such as Dermol 600® are similarly effective and much safer.

Cream based antibiotics

There are a number of creams available that contain antibiotics or a mixture of antibiotics and steroids. A number of these products contain an antibiotic called Fusidic acid examples include Fucidin®, Fucidin-H® and Fucibet®. I rarely use these creams as in some areas the bacteria which infect eczema are now resistant to this antibiotic. They are also only available in a cream base and it is important to use ointment based products when treating eczema. There is less bacterial resistance to other cream based antibiotics such as Trimovate®. Creams containing antiseptics such as Betnovate-C® and Timodine® are probably a better choice. I still though rarely use these as all cream based antibiotics can cause allergic reactions. Most dermatologists agree that it is best to treat infections with tablet/syrup antibiotics rather than cream antibiotics.

Treating bacterial infections

If you suspect that your child may have infected eczema you must seek an urgent opinion from a healthcare professional. In general infected eczema does not respond to cream based antibiotics and tablet or syrup preparations are required. In most cases your doctor will prescribe a penicillin based antibiotic called Flucloxacillin, this antibiotic tends to be both effective and is safe when given to children. It is taken four times a day and the dose will depend on the age and weight of your child. Other commonly used antibiotics include Erythromycin and Clarithromycin. It is important to stop using steroids and steroid alternatives such as Protopic® when eczema is infected. These creams will stop your child's immune system fighting the infection. Once your child has taken antibiotics for two to three days it is normally safe to reintroduce steroids and steroid alternatives, although you should always follow the advice of your healthcare professional.

Eczema Herpeticum

Eczema herpeticum is very serious condition, if you suspect your child may have it then you must seek immediate medical attention. In eczema herpeticum the child's eczema becomes infected with the virus that causes cold sores, the Herpes Simplex virus. It leads to a very rapid deterioration of eczema which will get worse over hours, this compares to bacterial infection which in which the eczema worsens over days. Within the eczema you will see many small ulcers a few millimeters wide which are often grouped together, you may also see tiny blisters. Like with bacterial infection it is important to stop using steroids and steroid alternatives such as Protopic® while eczema is infected. Doctors will treat eczema herpeticum with a combination of an antiviral medicine and an antibiotic as there is often bacterial infection alongside the viral infection. Some children require hospitalisation whilst being treated and it is particularly important to seek medical attention if the infection is near the eyes.

Allergy and Eczema

Key points

- There are few areas in medicine more argued about controversial than the relationship between eczema and allergy

- One thing which is agreed upon is that this is very complicated area in which we only have a limited understanding

- Most cases of eczema are not directly caused by allergy, nor are most flares of eczema caused by allergic reactions

- Children with eczema are more likely to have food and other allergies

- There is no good allergy test available which can tell us if a particular food or chemical is making a child's eczema worse

- There are only a very small number of children whose eczema is worsened by food allergy and improve with exclusion diets

Eczema and allergy

The number of cases of eczema worldwide has been rising dramatically, particularly in the developed world. There are many theories for this, one of which is that children are being exposed to allergens which are causing the eczema. Allergens are compounds that cause allergic reactions, the most common of which are house dust mites, pollen and pet fur. As well as eczema they are thought to be triggers for asthma and hayfever. Often children with eczema have asthma and hayfever and this is due to a combination of genetic atopy and exposure to allergens.

This brings up two important questions. If we can prevent exposure of very young children to allergens will it stop them developing eczema? And if we can prevent children who have eczema being exposed to allergens will it make them better? Sadly we simply do not know the answer to these questions although there are a lot of researchers trying their best to find the answers for us.

There is also a point about practicality. It may be relatively easy prevent your child coming in contact with pets, but it is nearly impossible to eliminate house dust mite and pollen. Parents sometimes ask me if they should get rid of their pet to help their child's eczema. This is a question I cannot answer as even if your child has a proven pet fur allergy, removing the pet will not necessarily make the child's eczema better. Similarly I am asked by parents if they should remove all the carpets in the house to reduce house dust mite levels. Nearly all people with eczema are allergic to house dust mite but removing all the carpets in house may or may not help with a child's eczema. What on the outside seems fairly simple is actually frustratingly complicated.

Food allergies

Parents often suspect that allergies to foods have either caused their child's eczema or are leading to flares of eczema. In fact there is little research evidence that food allergy has any role in eczema. To complicate matters children with eczema are more likely to have food allergies. When children have food allergy and are exposed to the food in question it causes symptoms such as stomach upset or swelling of the lips rather than flaring eczema. The whole subject is made even more difficult as there is not an accurate test for diagnosing if a food is causing eczema to flare.

The only effective way to see if certain foods are affecting your child's eczema is to keep a food diary. A particular food needs to be excluded for at least 6 weeks and then reintroduced to see if it has an effect on the eczema. It is particularly important to only exclude foods after discussion with a healthcare professional. I have seen a number of children become deficient in essential vitamins and minerals with exclusion diets and this in itself can cause flares of eczema. If you are excluding more than one food group you should consult a dietician or healthcare professional to check it is safe to do so.

The few times I have seen a true food allergy causing eczema have all been in children under one year of age at the time of weaning. They have presented with very severe eczema all over their skin when food has been introduced into the diet. For these children allergy testing is useful and is best done a doctor who specialises in allergy. The most common food allergies are to eggs, cow's milk, peanuts, soy and wheat.

Allergy testing

What we want is an allergy test that will tell us that when your child is exposed to a particular allergen then the eczema will flare and ultimately when you exclude that allergen the eczema will get better. Unfortunately this test does not exist. There are many charlatans that claim this test does exist and they will happily take large amounts of your money to do these tests. I can assure you if this test did exist then I would be using it every day and I would be telling you about it in this book.

There are many types of allergy and various allergy tests for these particular conditions. When these allergy tests are used incorrectly in children with eczema the results are unreliable and unhelpful. Sometimes doctors send a blood allergy test called specific IgE or a RAST test. This type of allergy test is not helpful in children with bad eczema and gives many untrue positive results. Prick testing is another type of allergy testing where a tiny needle is used to introduce allergens into the skin, normally on the forearm. Like with RAST testing there are often positive results that have little or nothing to do with the eczema.

Many children with eczema have allergies but these are unrelated to their eczema. Asthma and hayfever are both more common in children with eczema and allergies related to these or other conditions will make allergy tests positive. With current tests it is simply impossible to distinguish which allergies are relevant to which conditions. For these reasons I do not routinely undertake allergy testing for children with eczema.

Should I forget about allergy?

I like to take a pragmatic and practical approach to treating eczema. I have found that parents who actively seek out allergy testing and try to find allergic causes of their child's eczema often do not succeed and find the process frustrating. As the majority of eczema is not due to allergies or is due to allergens that cannot be excluded it is reasonable to argue that there is little benefit in doing this. I council parents that they should put all their efforts into treatment, applying the creams is not particularly nice but it is effective and if done properly it will make your child better. In all my years of practice I have yet to come across a child who has been able to cure their eczema by excluding particular foods from their diet.

What if all treatments fail

The most common reason for treatment failing is that treatment is not being done correctly. It is not due to lack of effort but often parents are led astray by poor advice from the internet and even from healthcare professionals. By following the advice in this book you should be able to identify what you can do to improve the treatment you are giving your child.

The most common reasons I see for children not getting better are:

- Not using a topical steroid. Often parents are scared of using steroids and simply do not want to use them on their children. I have hopefully reassured you that steroids are safe when used properly and using them is the key to making eczema better.

- Using the wrong steroid. Often non-specialist healthcare professionals are not confident when prescribing steroids and will give inappropriately weak preparations. Please read and follow the advice I have given on which steroids to use and if you are unsure take expert advice from a dermatologist.

- Using the wrong steroid preparation. Well over half the children I see in clinic are prescribed steroid creams by their family doctors. In nearly all cases of eczema steroid ointments should be used, not creams. This small change can make a big difference.

- Not using enough steroids. Both parents and family doctors are reluctant to use steroids and try and use as little as possible. When eczema is bad it needs steroids to be both applied and applied in appropriate quantities. A headache will not get better with a quarter a tablet of paracetamol and neither will eczema get better with a tiny amount of steroid. In unsure then rely on the finger tip unit method.

- Not using steroids regularly. Again and again I see health professionals prescribing short courses of steroids to be stopped after a few days. Eczema is a chronic condition, it is not going to be cured in a week and it will flare when steroids are stopped. Use steroids regularly, every day to treat the eczema and stop it flaring.

- Using the wrong moisturiser. Every day I see parents who tell me the same story, the moisturiser they use works, but within a few minutes the skin is dry again. This is because the moisturiser it too thin, if this is happening you need a greasy ointment to keep the moisture in the skin. Moisturisers need to be used all over, at least twice a day and in surprisingly large quantities.

- Using soaps, bubble baths or shampoos. Parents are targeted by marketing campaigns promoting soaps which are claimed to be good for the skin or designed for children. All soaps, shampoos, bubble baths and shower gels are bad for children with eczema and need to be avoided. Use your moisturiser as a soap substitute.

- Not treating infections properly. Some healthcare professionals still favor cream based antibiotics rather than tablets/syrup. In your child has weepy, infected eczema then they need tablets/syrup antibiotics. For bad infections the steroids need to be stopped for a few days whilst the antibiotics work.

In my specialist clinic I see children who have had eczema for years and have seen numerous healthcare professionals including other specialists yet in nearly all cases they are making the same simple mistakes as described above. By reading this book and following the advice I have given 99% of children will get better. I cannot emphasise enough how important it is to get the basics right.

There are though a very small minority of children with eczema who do not respond to treatment even when everything is being done right. Most of these children have very severe atopic eczema and need treatment with strong steroid ointments under the close supervision of a doctor. In very severe, treatment resistant cases of eczema dermatologists may use other treatments such as phototherapy and medications that suppress the immune system. There are also a small number of exceptionally rare genetic and nutritional conditions that can mimic eczema. If you have a child that is not improving despite following the advice of your healthcare professional and what is written in this book then you should request to see a dermatologist.

Appendix: Commonly Used Creams in Eczema

Moisturisers

Brand Name	Notes
Aquadrate® Cream	Cream based moisturiser with 10% urea
Aqueous Cream	None branded product, see notes of aqueous cream in section on moisturisers
Aveeno® Cream Aveeno® Lotion	Available in lotion and cream preparation, contains oatmeal. Aveeno® produce a large extended range of additional products
Balneum® Plus Cream	Cream based moisturiser with 5% urea and 3% lauromacrogols
Calmurid® Cream	Cream based moisturiser with 10% urea and 5% lactic acid
Cetraben® Cream Cetraben® Lotion	Medium greasy cream and thinner lotion are available
Dermamist® Spray	Spray on moisturiser
Dermol® Cream Dermol® 500 lotion	Cream and Lotion based moisturisers which contain antiseptics
Diprobase® Cream Diprobase® Ointment Diprobase® Lotion	Available in a cream form and a greasy ointment
Doublebase® Gel Doublebase® Dayleve Gel Doublebase Wash	Gel is a light moisturiser that rubs in easily and leaves little shine on the skin. Dayleve is a little greasier and lasts longer. Wash is in a pump dispenser to use a soap substitute
E45® Lotion E45® Cream E45® Emollient Wash Cream E45® Itch relief	Available in cream and lotion preparations. The emollient wash is in a pump dispenser to be used as a soap substitute. E45® itch relief has 5% urea and 3% macrogol lauryl ether. E45® produce a large extended range of additional products
Eczmol® Cream	Cream based moisturiser with antiseptic
Emollin® Spray	Spray on moisturiser
Emulsifying Ointment	None branded product, designed as a soap substitute can also be used as a greasy moisturiser

Epaderm® Cream Epaderm® Ointment	Cream and ointment preparations are available
Eucerin® Intensive Cream	Cream based moisturiser with 10% urea
Hydromol® Cream Hydromol® Ointment Hydromol® Intensive	In addition to cream and ointment preparations, Hydromol® intensive contains 10% urea
Hydrous Ointment	None branded product, contains lanolin
Liquid & White Soft Paraffin Ointment	None branded product, also known as 'WSP 50/LP 50' or '50/50'. A very greasy ointment
Nutraplus® Cream	Cream based moisturiser with 10% urea
Oilatum® Cream Oilatum® junior Lotion Oilatum® junior Cream	Comes in cream and lotion preparations. The junior branded products are the same as the adult products
QV® Cream QV® Lotion QV® Intensive Ointment	Available in lotion, cream and ointment preparations
Ultrabase® Cream	Cream based moisturiser
Unguentum M® Cream	Cream based moisturiser
ZeroAQS® Cream	Cream based moisturiser, similar to Aqueous cream
Zerobase® Cream	Cream based moisturiser, similar in consistency to Diprobase® Cream
Zerocream® Cream	Cream based moisturiser
Zeroderm® Ointment	Ointment, similar in consistency to Epaderm® Ointment
Zeroguent® Cream	Cream based moisturiser, similar consistency to Unguentum M® Cream

Bath and Shower Moisturisers

Brand Name	Notes
Alpha Keri Bath®	Bath oil
Aveeno® Bath and Shower Oil Aveeno® Colloidal	Contains oatmeal. Oil can be diluted in bath water or used in the shower. Colloidal powder can be dissolved in the bath
Balneum® Bath Oil	Bath oil, contains soya

Cetraben® Emollient Bath Additive	Oil can be diluted in bath water or used in the shower
Dermalo® Bath Emollient	Bath oil
Dermol® 200 Shower Emollient Dermol® 600 Bath Emollient	Shower product comes in a hooked showergel like container and contains antiseptic. Bath oil contains antiseptic
Diprobath® Bath Additive	Bath oil
Doublebase® Bath Doublebase® Shower	Bath product is an oil to be diluted in the bath. Shower product comes in a hooked showergel like container to be used as a soap substitute in the shower
E45® Emollient Bath Oil E45® Emollient Shower Cream	Bath product is an oil to be diluted in the bath. Shower product can be used as a soap substitute in the shower
Emulsiderm® Liquid Emulsion	Bath oil with antiseptic
Hydromol® Bath & Shower Emollient	Oil can be diluted in bath water or used in the shower
Imuderm® Bath Oil	Bath oil, contains almond oil
Oilatum® Shower gel Oilatum® junior Bath Oilatum® Bath Oilatum® Plus Bath additive	Oils can be diluted in the bath, shower gel is a soap substitute for the shower. Oilatum plus contains antiseptics
QV® Bath Oil	Oil can be diluted in bath water or used in the shower
Zerolatum® Emollient Bath Additive	Bath oil with similar ingredients to Oilatum®
Zeroneum® Emollient Bath Additive	Bath oil with similar ingredients to Balneum®

Steroids

Brand Name	Steroid Name	Notes
Alphaderm®	Hydrocortisone 1%; Cream	Mild strength steroid + 10% urea
Aureocort®	Triamcinolone acetonide 0.1%; Ointment	Potent strength steroid + antibiotic
Betamethasone Valerate	Betamethasone Valerate 0.1%, 0.025%; Cream & Ointment	0.1% is a Potent strength steroid, 0.025% is a Moderate strength steroid
Betacap®	Betamethasone Valerate 0.1%; Scalp Application	Potent strength steroid
Betnovate®	Betamethasone Valerate 0.1%; Cream, Ointment, Lotion & Scalp Application	Potent strength steroid
Betnovate-C®	Betamethasone Valerate 0.1%; Cream & Ointment	Potent strength steroid + antiseptic
Betnovate-N®	Betamethasone Valerate 0.1%; Cream & Ointment	Potent strength steroid + antibiotic
Betnovate-RD®	Betamethasone Valerate 0.025%; Cream & Ointment	Moderate strength steroid
Bettamousse®	Betamethasone Valerate 0.1%; Foam	Potent strength steroid
Calmurid HC®	Hydrocortisone 1%; Cream	Mild strength steroid + 1% urea + 10% lactic acid
Canesten HC®	Hydrocortisone 1%; Cream	Mild strength steroid + anti-fungal
Clobetasone Butyrate	Clobetasone Butyrate 0.05%; Cream & Ointment	Moderate strength steroid
Clobetasol Propionate	Clobetasol Propionate 0.05%; Cream & Ointment	Very potent strength steroid
Cutivate®	Fluticasone Propionate 0.05%; Cream & Ointment	Potent strength steroid
Daktacort®	Hydrocortisone 1%; Cream & Ointment	Mild strength steroid + anti-fungal
Dermovate®	Clobetasol Propionate 0.05%; Cream, Scalp	Very potent strength steroid

	Application & Ointment	
Dioderm®	Hydrocortisone 0.1%; Cream	Very weak steroid cream
Diprosalic®	Betamethasone Diproprinate 0.05%; Ointment & Scalp application	Potent strength steroid + Salicylic acid
Diprosone®	Betamethasone Diproprinate 0.05%; Cream, Ointment & Lotion	Potent strength steroid
Elocon®	Mometasone furoate 0.1%; Cream, Ointment & Scalp Application	Potent strength steroid
Eumovate®	Clobetasone Butyrate 0.05%; Cream & Ointment	Moderate strength steroid
Eurax-Hydrocortisone®	Hydrocortisone 0.25%; Cream	Very weak steroid cream + 10% crotamiton
Fucidin H®	Hydrocortisone 1%; Cream & Ointment	Mild strength steroid + antibiotic
Fucibet®	Betamethasone Valerate 0.1%; Cream & Lipid Cream	Potent strength steroid + antibiotic
Haelan®	Fludroxycortide 0.0125%; Cream, Ointment & Tape	Moderate strength steroid
Hydrocortisone	Hydrocortisone 0.5%, 1% & 2.5%; Cream & Ointment	Mild strength steroid
Locoid®	Hydrocortisone Butyrate 0.1%; Cream, Lipocream, Scalp lotion & Ointment	Potent strength steroid
Locoid Crelo®	Hydrocortisone Butyrate 0.1%; Lotion	Potent strength steroid
Lotriderm®	Betamethasone Valerate 0.1%; Cream	Potent strength steroid + antifungal
Metosyn®	Fluocinonide 0.05%; Cream & Ointment	Potent strength steroid
Mildison®	Hydrocortisone 1%; Lipocream	Mild strength steroid

Modrasone®	Alcometasone Dipropionate 0.05%; Cream & Ointment	Moderate strength steroid
Nerisone®	Diflucortolone Valerate 0.1%; Cream, Oily Cream & Ointment	Potent strength steroid
Nerisone forte®	Diflucortolone Valerate 0.3%; Oily Cream & Ointment	Very potent strength steroid
Nystaform-HC®	Hydrocortisone 0.5%, 1%; Cream & Ointment	Mild strength steroid + anti-fungal + antiseptic
Synalar®	Fluocinolone acetonide 0.025%; Cream, Gel & Ointment	Potent strength steroid
Synalar C®	Fluocinolone acetonide 0.025%; Cream, Ointment	Potent strength steroid + antiseptic
Synalar N®	Fluocinolone acetonide 0.025%; Cream, Ointment	Potent strength steroid + antibiotic
Synalar 1 in 4 Dilution®	Fluocinolone acetonide 0.00625%; Cream & Ointment	Moderate strength steroid
Synalar 1 in 10 Dilution®	Fluocinolone acetonide 0.0025%; Cream	Mild strength steroid
Timodine®	Hydrocortisone 0.5%; Cream	Mild strength steroid + anti-fungal + antiseptic
Trimovate®	Clobetasone Butyrate 0.05%; Cream	Moderate strength steroid + antibiotic + antifungal
Ultralanum Plain®	Fluocortolone 0.25%; Cream & Ointment	Moderate strength steroid